A Natural Guide to Prediabetes

Syndrome X and Metabolic Syndrome

Martin Stone, M.H.

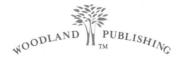

WOODLAND PUBLISHING
TM

For permissions, ordering information, or bulk quantity discounts, please contact: Woodland Publishing, 448 East 800 North, Orem, Utah 84097
Visit our Web site: www.woodlandpublishing.com
Toll-free number: (800) 777-2665

Cataloging-in-Publication data available from the Library of Congress.

ISBN-13: 978-1-58054-465-8
ISBN-10: 1-58054-465-7

Printed in the United States of America

06   07   08   09   10   1   2   3   4   5   6   7   8   9   10

Contents

Pre-Diabetes, Syndrome X, and Metabolic Syndrome

Prediabetes, Syndrome X, and metabolic syndrome—including insulin resistance—occurs when there is a higher-than-normal level of fasting insulin that is associated with an increased risk of developing type 2 diabetes. Hyperinsulinemia often predates diabetes by several years. You can have this condition for decades in some cases but your doctor often will not treat it because your blood sugar is still mostly within the high normal range.

Hyperinsulinemia is an endocrine disorder characterized by a failure of our blood-sugar control system (BSCS) to work properly. It manifests when insulin progressively loses its effectiveness in helping blood glucose enter into the sixty-seven trillion or so cells that make up our bodies. Insulin levels in the blood rapidly rise to damaging levels and, together with the resulting elevated glucose levels, account for much of the damage to our arteries and vascular system. This loss of effectiveness is not due to any change in the insulin produced by the pancreas. It is due to a change in the cellular metabolism of almost every cell in our body. Our cells no longer recognize or react to insulin as they should.

Our blood-sugar control system works to maintain our blood sugar at a predetermined set point. This set point is important because high levels of blood glucose can damage our blood vessels. We need enough insulin to keep our blood sugar below this threshold, but insulin levels can't be too high either. High levels of insulin will also cause blood vessel damage.

A properly functioning blood-sugar control system will automatically maintain correct blood-sugar levels under all circumstances—whether we have eaten a meal or have been fasting for a week.

It has been theorized that as insulin becomes progressively less effective, the pancreas starts to produce more insulin in an attempt to control blood-sugar levels. As a result, the pancreas has to perform beyond its intended design. This over-production of insulin by the pancreas is a direct result of improperly functioning cells that no longer recognize insulin produced in the body and is the root cause of Syndrome X.

In either event, type 2 diabetes is diagnosed at this point if the individual is lucky. Remember, the majority of diabetics and prediabetics are not discovered until the disease is fully developed. Of course, hyperinsulinemia has been active for some while, often for a long while, by the time the diagnosis is made. About 41 million people in the United States, ages forty to seventy-four, have prediabetes (hyperinsulinemia). Recent research has shown that some long-term damage to the body, especially the heart and circulatory system, may occur during the prediabetes years.

As many as one in four American adults and 40 percent of adults age forty or older have metabolic syndrome, an increase of 61 percent over the last decade. Some medical professionals question its existence as a distinct medical condition, and say more research is needed. In the meantime, an epidemic is starting that can be easily prevented; the first step is recognizing that there is a problem.

Whether or not medical researchers agree, metabolic syndrome is a growing health problem in the United States and worldwide, according to a new scientific statement by the American Heart Association and National Heart, Lung, and Blood Institute.

The statement, published in *Circulation: Journal of the American Heart Association,* confirmed the recommendations on metabolic syndrome of the National Cholesterol Education Program (NCEP) Adult Treatment Panel III (ATP III) report made in 2001, with some modifications.

Metabolic syndrome, which consists of multiple interrelated risk factors, increases the risk for atherosclerotic cardiovascular disease up to three times and raises the risk for type 2 diabetes by up to five times. It affects over 25 percent of the adult population in America, which translates to over seventy million Americans.

Blood tests are not the only method of diagnosing metabolic syndrome. There are physical signs and changes that are easily recognizable.

The criteria for metabolic syndrome include:

- Elevated waist circumference (abdominal obesity)
- Elevated triglycerides
- Reduced high-density lipoprotein cholesterol (HDL-C or "good" cholesterol)
- Elevated blood pressure
- Elevated fasting glucose

An individual who meets three of these criteria has metabolic syndrome.

Metabolic syndrome isn't a disease in the same way as the flu or dysentery; it is a cluster of disorders affecting your body's metabolism. They include high blood pressure, high insulin levels, excess body weight, and abnormal cholesterol levels. All of these conditions contribute to varying degrees to your likelihood of developing diabetes, heart disease, or stroke. Each of these disorders is by itself a risk factor for other diseases. In combination, though, these disorders dramatically boost your chances of developing potentially life-threatening illnesses.

Are the predisposing physical characteristics of metabolic syndrome the same as in diabetes?

Do you have metabolic syndrome or are you at risk of developing it? Take this questionnaire.

- Are you overweight by 20 to 30 percent?
- Do you get less than thirty minutes of exercise per day?
- Is your blood pressure elevated even slightly? (130/80 or higher)
- Is there a family history of diabetes?
- Did you develop gestational diabetes during pregnancy or did you deliver a baby that weighed more than nine pounds?
- Are you African American, Native American, Hispanic, or Asian American/Pacific Islander?

If you answered yes to any of these questions, you are at a greater than average risk of developing Syndrome X or diabetes. If you answered yes to more than two of these criteria, you almost certainly have metabolic syndrome or are very close to it.

One study reported that men who had three symptoms of metabolic syndrome are twice as likely to have a cardiovascular event such as stroke or heart attack and are three times as likely to develop heart disease as those who don't. It also reported that males who reported four or five criteria had four times the risk of heart attack and stroke, and twenty-four times the risk of developing full-blown diabetes.

Not surprisingly, a research study initiated by Johns Hopkins University reported that physical exercise improves physical fitness in people aged fifty-five to seventy-five and reduces the occurrence of symptoms or risk factors for heart disease and metabolic syndrome. There was a reported 23 percent reduction in cardiac events such as stroke or heart attack, which was associated with a reduced fat layer and increased lean muscle tissue rather than the improved fitness level of the participants.

In almost all cases, Syndrome X and metabolic syndrome occur before diabetes. Unfortunately it is mostly undiagnosed and unrecognized, which can lead to preventable cases of diabetes.

How does diet contribute to Syndrome X, metabolic syndrome, and type 2 diabetes?

Carbohydrates are primarily found in grains, flours, sugars, and fruits. They're found in other foods as well, but these are the primary forms. When we eat high-carbohydrate foods, they are eventually converted to glucose, a sugar that the body uses for energy production on the cellular level.

In order for cells to utilize glucose as an energy source, the glucose must be able to enter the cells. This is where insulin, which is produced by the pancreas, plays its role. Insulin's function is to help create a gateway into the cell, allowing the glucose to enter and start the process of cellular metabolism.

Diabetics or prediabetics can't utilize these blood sugars because they don't produce insulin or the insulin they do produce is not recognized by the body. Either way this causes blood-sugar levels to increase.

In non-diabetics, blood sugar that is not used immediately goes through various processes that allow it to be stored as fats in the body for use at a future time. In diabetics, not only are the sugars not utilized by the cells or stored as fats, they are removed from the blood and secreted in the urine. Sugar levels in urine are still used as a primary tool to diagnose diabetes. If left untreated, the end result of diabetes is steady weight loss eventually leading to death.

When the body's metabolism and pancreas are functioning

correctly, simple carbohydrates or sugars such as a candy bar will enter into the bloodstream very rapidly, which forces the pancreas to secrete substantial levels of insulin that allows glucose into the cells through insulin receptors in the cell walls. When simple carbohydrates such as sugar are eaten, this rise in blood sugar is even faster because these simple sugars have no fiber, minerals, or other nutrients to control and slow the sugar's entry into the bloodstream.

Blood sugar is used in three ways:

1. About 50 percent is used for immediate energy
2. About 10 percent is stored in the muscle and liver as glycogen
3. Approximately 40 percent is stored as fats, triglycerides, and cholesterol

Long-Term Complications

Cardiovascular disease is one of the primary conditions associated with diabetes and blood-sugar disorders in general. As mentioned earlier, diabetics are two to four times more likely to develop cardiovascular disease than the rest of the general population. Cardiovascular disease manifests itself in several different ways, including heart attack, stroke, angina, atherosclerosis and arteriosclerosis.

One of the current theories as to how damage occurs to the inner lining of blood vessels (called the intima), involves high sugar and insulin levels in the blood that creates a caustic reaction to this delicate inner layer similar to an acid burn. Some also believe that a chemical change occurs in diabetics that allows blood vessels to become more vulnerable to this kind of damage.

Arteries of newborn babies are like glass, smooth with no irregularities. When high levels of insulin come in contact with the interior walls of the arteries, it has a caustic or acidic effect on the tissue, inflaming the area and creating the initial injury that causes plaque to accumulate as a sort of bandage.

As this caustic damage continues year after year and as

the cholesterol plaque increases as a result, a reduction in the inner diameter of the blood vessels starts to occur, resulting in increased blood pressure as a result of the restricted blood flow. This is similar to stepping on a garden hose and forcing the water to only trickle out.

Arterial plaque in blood vessels is called arteriosclerosis or hardening of the arteries and is the root cause of most cardiovascular disease. Left untreated, this narrowing of the blood vessels forces your heart to work harder to pump enough blood and oxygen to your body's organs and tissues thereby creating higher pressure and more damage to arteries and arterioles, the very small arteries that connect larger arteries to tiny capillaries.

A secondary consideration is the fact that as a result of poor circulation to all the organs and tissues of the body, reduced function in all areas of the body will eventually occur, further impacting the overall health of the individual.

In addition, plaque may dislodge from the sides of the artery wall, forming a blockage in another part of the body causing a heart attack or stroke.

Does the increased incidence of Syndrome X and metabolic syndrome have anything to do with the standard American diet (SAD)?

A large-scale Harvard Medical School study monitored 52,000 nurses and their pattern of consumption of soft drinks and sugary fruit cocktails over eight years. This study reported that consumption of as little as one non-diet soda per day was enough to increase weight gain and the risk of type 2 diabetes in comparison to individuals who drink less than one non-diet soda a month.

Most of us know that consuming sugar, especially in the high amounts that are found in soft drinks, can lead to obesity and unhealthy weight gain. Nevertheless, both Coca-Cola and Pepsi and the American Beverage Association (ABA), a soft-drink lobbyist group, have all pointed out that both the American Diabetes Association and the National Institutes of Health have not specifically associated consumption of soft drinks with the onset of diabetes. Despite the fact that the ABA has stated that the real cause of diabetes is obesity and that individuals who drink large amounts of soda often have other unhealthy habits, the fact remains that each twelve-ounce bottle of soda contains ten teaspoons of sugar.

The obesity link is there—fully 80 percent of people with type 2 diabetes are obese. It doesn't take a rocket scientist to realize that high sugar consumption leads to obesity, which can then lead to diabetes.

So the question is: Does obesity cause diabetes or does eating a diet high in simple carbohydrates, including sugar, result in obesity, a prediabetic condition and eventual diabetes if left to run its normal course?

Which comes first, the chicken or the egg?

Scientists at the Eleanor Roosevelt Institute at the University of Denver have made a revolutionary discovery that for the first time establishes a biochemical connection between obesity and type 2 diabetes. This study was published in the *Journal of Endocrinology*.

This study of mice reported that in order for obese mice to develop diabetes, melanocyte stimulating hormone (MSH), which is made by the POMC (proopiomelanocortin) gene that is found in both mice and humans, needs to be present.

Obese mice without MSH did not develop diabetes, but with the administration of MSH blood-sugar levels and increased insulin resistance were observed. A reasonable conclusion could be that this specific hormone could play a role in the development of type 2 diabetes. This study may lead to more accurate prediction and testing procedures for individuals who are genetically predisposed due to family histories of blood-sugar disorders such as diabetes.

In addition, overeating stresses the insides of individual cells. Stress occurs in the endoplasmic reticulum (ER) found inside every cell in the body when we overeat. When the ER is exposed to more nutrients than it can handle, an alarm signal is sent out to the cell wall, which reduces the activity and receptiveness of insulin receptors. This in turn results in insulin resistance from frequent overeating, resulting in high levels of blood sugar, which is one of the early signs of diabetes or metabolic syndrome.

Metabolism and Insulin Resistance

Recent research has reported that not only do high blood-sugar levels create health problems, but also high insulin levels. Excessive insulin is related to cardiovascular disease and chronic inflammation throughout the body.

Insulin resistance is associated with obesity, high blood pressure, and type 2 diabetes, in addition to playing a major role in fat storage and cholesterol function.

It is also theorized that insulin resistance may have a link to reduced levels of HDL cholesterol and estrogen loss that commonly occur in women after menopause.

For this reason, it's always a good idea to eat foods that have a low to moderate reading on the glycemic index. What this translates to is eating as few simple carbohydrates and sugars as possible.

In the May 3, 2001, issue of the *New England Journal of Medicine*, a study reported that limitation of fat intake and increasing fiber along with increased exercise resulted in a 58 percent reduction in the development of diabetes. This human study included 522 overweight, middle-aged participants, which reflects the average North American who is at risk of developing diabetes.

A U.S. government–funded study that followed three thousand diabetes-prone individuals reported that simple changes in lifestyle, which included losing five to seven percent of total body weight and participating in thirty minutes of daily exercise also produced the same 58 percent reduction in diabetes risk.

This study was different in that it compared this strategy with the use of Metformin, a common pharmaceutical approach to diabetes management. The individuals in the study that only took Metformin reduced their risk by only 31 percent as compared to the 58 percent of the individuals that lost weight and exercised.

We know that eating carbohydrates to excess, especially simple carbohydrates, increases blood insulin levels in an attempt to regulate blood sugar, however research has reported that high-carbohydrate diets do not necessarily increase the risk of developing type 2 diabetes.

This research may be flawed despite the fact that researchers reported that high-sugar diets worsen glucose tolerance in non-diabetic animals and humans. The studies supposedly used high amounts of sugars in proportion to other foods normally found in the standard American diet. It is now believed that the researchers dramatically underestimated the amounts of sugars normally found in the current average diet. In the late nineteenth century, the average consumption of sugar was only five pounds per person per year; current estimated sugar consumption is 135 pounds per person per year. Interestingly, and perhaps coincidentally, cancer and cardiovascular disease were virtually nonexistent in the early twentieth century.

Or is it a coincidence?

An early diabetes study reported in increase in diabetes in a group of Yemenite Jews who changed their diet from eating no sugar to one that included sugar. This early study assumed that other factors such as weight gain contributed to the increase in diabetes. Once again, weight gain was seen as the primary culprit in diabetes development, which may have skewed the interpretation of the study.

Other studies have indicated that there was no correlation between high sugar intake and development of diabetes. One such study of one hundred diabetics took place in 1935. The researcher placed half the patients on a low-fat diet and the other half on a high-fat diet. The results astonished everyone, as the low-fat dieters were able to reduce blood cholesterol levels and the dosage of insulin by over 58 percent, and 24 percent of the participants eliminated their insulin completely while maintaining blood-sugar stability just as a non-diabetic person would.

The high-fat participants were not able to reduce their insulin dosage at all. The researcher theorized that the low-fat diet was the primary reason why the first group did not develop heart disease or other principal symptoms of diabetes, including gangrene. Unfortunately, with the advent of insulin use as the primary treatment for diabetes, it was then thought that diabetes could not be controlled by diet despite the fact that early diabetes treatment plans consisted solely of dietary restrictions.

A 1979 University of Kentucky Medical Center study required that participants eat one pound of sugar every day with the rest of the low-fat diet composed of only 5 percent fats. I know this is a shocking approach, but the results are even more shocking. After eleven weeks of eating one pound of sugar per day, not even one person became diabetic based on the glucose tolerance test and weekly blood-sugar-level evaluations; blood-sugar levels were always in the low range despite the fact that it was thought that sugar caused diabetes.

This same researcher then tried a high-fat diet consisting of 65 percent fat with almost no fiber and after several weeks every participant became diabetic. He tried the same approach again with a 45 percent fat diet with no complex carbohydrates or fiber and once again everyone tested diabetic.

A third study was initiated utilizing a diet comprised of 40 percent complex carbohydrates and 43 percent fat. Despite the fact that blood-sugar levels were higher than the group that ate the pound of sugar per day, these levels did not enter into the diabetic range. It is surmised that the vegetables and fruit fibers have a protective action on the insulin itself and may also reduce the speed that sugars enter the bloodstream.

The medical community, believing that obesity causes diabetes, often suggests that overweight diabetic patients lose weight in an attempt to eradicate this condition.

This approach was tested and reported in the May, 1980, edition of the *Medical Times*. Twenty lean diabetics were chosen to participate. They ate a 70 percent complex-carbohydrate, high-fiber diet for two weeks that included crackers, whole wheat, shredded wheat, beans, and raw fruit. It was reported that weight loss alone did not cure diabetes, although it did help to some degree. Interestingly, the same results as the 1935 study were reported with a 58 percent reduction in insulin use and a 30 percent cholesterol reduction.

We now know that high carbohydrate diet along with high-fat content dramatically increases the incidence of diabetes and that sugar or other carbohydrate foods temporarily raise blood sugar and the need for insulin.

There are two different types of carbohydrate foods: high glycemic and low glycemic. Many starchy foods like potatoes have a glycemic activity or index that is similar to table sugar. Consuming high amounts of these foods increases the risk of type 2 diabetes.

On the other hand, eating a diet high in carbohydrate-rich foods with low glycemic indices is associated with a low risk of type 2 diabetes. Beans, peas, most fruit, and oats have low glycemic indices, despite their high carbohydrate content, due mostly to the health-promoting effects of soluble fiber.

Until recently, health professionals have recommended sugar restriction to people with diabetes, even though short-term high-sugar diets have been shown not to cause blood-sugar problems in people with diabetes. Currently, the American Diabetic Association guidelines do not prohibit the use of moderate amounts of sugar, as long as the goals of normalizing blood levels of glucose, triglycerides, and cholesterol are being achieved.

Despite the ADA's dietary guidelines suggesting that moderate use of sugar is safe for diabetics, most medical doctors recommend at the minimum a reduction or elimination of sugar and junk foods containing sugars and fats and replacing them with high-fiber whole foods with a low glycemic index. One study suggested omega-3 fatty acids contained in fish, when combined with a weight-loss program, improved cholesterol and blood-glucose levels and regulated insulin metabolism. It is theorized that omega-3 fatty acids improve cell wall permeability allowing more effective entry and activity of insulin and glucose.

Acting on statistics that suggest vegetarians have a much lower risk of type 2 diabetes than the general population, nonvegetarian patients with diabetic nerve damage were put on a vegan diet with no meat, dairy, or eggs, resulting in the disappearance of pain in less than one week in seventeen of twenty-one people.

Increasing levels of monounsaturated oils however are good for diabetics; these oils once again may play a role in maintaining the health of cell walls throughout the body.

Unfortunately it is hard to get people to change dietary habits and replace them with better ones despite the fact that even adolescents with type 1 diabetes exhibited better control over blood sugar and cholesterol with the addition of monounsaturated fats into the diet. The easiest way to incorporate monounsaturates into the diet is to use olive oil.

Worldwide Nutrition Trends

As of 1996, there has been a 30 percent increase in the consumption of calories from sugars, with fifty-four calories coming from soft drinks and thirteen calories coming from sugar-containing fruit drinks. According to the U.S. Department of Agriculture, the consumption of soft drinks has increased 500 percent in the last fifty years.

The continued increase in sugar and fat consumption has prompted the World Health Organization (WHO) to develop a report on diet to address the increasing problem of chronic diseases worldwide and develop a strategy to combat the problem.

The report contains scientific evidence on the relationship of diet, nutrition, and physical activity to chronic diseases such as diabetes, obesity, cancer, and cardiovascular disease.

This report came to the common-sense conclusion that a diet low in saturated fat, sugars, and salt and high in vegetables and fruit, along with regular physical activity will help to combat chronic disease.

Imagine that! Who knew?

The fact that one of the most prestigious and conservative health organizations in the world has come out against sugar consumption should give us pause. Chronic diseases are rapidly increasing. In 2001, about 59 percent of total deaths worldwide were due to chronic diseases, which make up 46 percent of diseases globally. Poor nutrition globally with decreasing exercise levels and higher levels of high-calorie, low-nutrition foods or empty calories are creating a higher incidence of chronic disease. Despite the fact that huge amounts of money are invested in North American health care, cardiovascular disease, cancer, and obesity are still the leading causes of death in North America and are now becoming major health issues around the world.

The authors note that even modest, population-wide changes in diet and physical activity can produce significant changes to the overall burden of chronic disease in a short time period. These are some of the recommendations:

- Fat intake should only be between 15 and 30 percent of total daily energy intake, with saturated fats being less than 10 percent
- Carbohydrate intake should be between 55 and 75 percent of daily intake
- Added sugars should be less than 10 percent of daily intake
- Daily intake of salt, which should be iodized, should be less than 5 grams a day

- Intake of fruit and vegetables should be at least 400 grams a day
- Protein should account for 10 percent to 15 percent of total daily intake
- Moderate-intensity activity for one hour each day, for most days of the week, is needed to maintain a healthy body weight

While these recommendations sound effective, the sugar industry is trying to block the implementation of this plan.

The U.S. Soft Drink Association has already come out against this report, which has concluded that sweetened drinks contribute to obesity. The USSDA is seeking to convince the government and public that we should not limit our sugar intake to less than 10 percent of our daily energy intake.

Now the U.S.-based Sugar Association is trying to get the report withdrawn (along with six other major food industry groups including the U.S. Council for International Business, of which Coca-Cola and Pepsico are a part), saying that up to 25 percent of our daily intake can come from sugar.

The sugar industry is threatening to lobby congress to cut off funding to the World Heath Organization unless WHO withdraws their report.

Amazing but true, this revelation has brought to the forefront the need for self-responsibility and education in health care. The attitude shown by these giants in the food (I use this word guardedly) industry is reminiscent of the attitude shown to the public by the tobacco industry. Remember? Apparently smoking was not that bad for you and didn't cause cancer.

The increase of sugar/fat use worldwide isn't the only issue concerning our health and diabetes. Soil conditions also play a major role.

Mineral Depletion

Data compiled by the USDA shows that at least 40 percent of people consume a diet that contains only 60 percent of the RDA (recommended daily allowance) of ten selected nutrients. This means that half or more of the population is clinically deficient in at least one important nutrient. The United States Food and Nutrition Board instituted RDAs over forty-five years ago. They were considered then as a standard for the amount of vitamins and minerals needed by a healthy person. We know now that RDAs only provide the bare minimum required to stop the signs of clinical malnutrition, such as scurvy, beriberi, and pellagra. New studies have shown since that substantially larger amounts help our bodies to work more efficiently.

Nutritionists would have us believe that it is possible for everyone to receive everything they need from a balanced diet. All this may be able to do is stop us from having obvious symptoms of certain nutritional deficiencies. There's a big difference between this and having the levels of nutrients needed in order to have excellent health. Why is it unlikely that we would be able to get the proper levels of nutrients needed in order to maintain our health from food alone?

Not only are the soils stripped of most mineral content, we now have irradiation of food and genetic manipulation of seed stocks to contend with. By the time foods get to market, most of the water-soluble vitamins have been oxidized and are gone. Our water is contaminated, as is our air.

At this point I would like to state that natural treatment of diabetes is a gradual process and uses a substantially different direction than drug treatment. Although prescription drug treatment for diabetes is very quick acting, it does nothing to normalize the body's production or secretion of insulin and does little to help normalize cell use of blood sugar.

While more gradual, natural treatments of diabetes, when successful, facilitate and normalize pancreatic action while decreasing cellular insulin resistance and optimizing blood-glucose levels. At the very least, this method of treatment can reduce the need for diabetic drug therapy while improving overall health through supplement use and dietary strategies.

Primary Antidiabetic Supplements

Chromium

Chromium is a micro-mineral that at one time was found in soils in almost every region of the world. The general population received enough chromium through diet up until the last fifty years, however with the advent of modern agriculture with its use of pesticides and chemical additives such as fertilizers in combination with consistent overuse and exhaustion of soils due to the need for high yields, chromium and other crucial minerals have been gradually depleted. Some of these other crucial minerals include magnesium, manganese, copper, calcium, and zinc. The end result is that vegetables and grains grown in these mineral-deficient soils are also mineral deficient.

You may ask why this is of importance. Chromium deficiency in the general population is probably one of the most health-affecting mineral deficiencies in not only the developed world but in those countries with naturally chromium-deficient soils such as Asia.

Our ability to absorb minerals and nutrients declines as we age. It is estimated that a fifty-year-old individual can absorb less than half of the calcium that an eighteen-year-old can. According to one expert, most individuals twenty or older are deficient in chromium and as a result age more quickly than they would if they had adequate supplies.

In addition, individuals with sedentary lifestyles, as well as athletes, both have a higher than usual risk of chromium deficiency. Chromium deficiency is also associated with pregnancy, stress, and complex thinking; in other words, anyone who lives an average life that uses even moderate amounts of sugars for metabolism or muscle fuel.

When a person is deficient in chromium, insulin does not function properly, which in turn can result in potentially dangerous levels of blood sugar and insulin. Does this sound familiar? It sounds like prediabetes to me.

Although chromium deficiency may be a primary reason in triggering diabetes, researchers do not believe that chromium deficiency is the primary underlying cause; therefore chromium supplements are not able to cure diabetes.

Nonetheless, because chromium significantly influences insulin levels and utilization, persons who have been diagnosed as having diabetes or are considered at risk of diabetes are strongly advised to consult with their health-care professional regarding chromium supplementation.

Recent research has reported that chromium improves blood-sugar levels in individuals with a variety of blood-sugar disorders, including type 1 and type 2 diabetes, metabolic syndrome, gestational diabetes, and steroid-induced diabetes.

One benefit of chromium supplementation has been manifested in over ten studies as a reduced need for insulin in type 1 diabetics to control blood-sugar levels. This is hypothesized to be the result of increased sensitivity to insulin by the cells.

You don't have to have diabetes or prediabetes to reap the benefits of chromium supplementation, because it will reduce cholesterol and triglycerides that contribute to heart disease.

Although several chromium studies reported little or no benefit from chromium use, all of these trials used 200 micrograms or less, which is not adequate to substantially affect blood-sugar levels, especially if it is a poorly absorbed form.

Although 200 micrograms of chromium per day is a typical dosage used in many blood-glucose studies, a more effective dose would be 500 to 1,000 micrograms per day for people with full-blown diabetes.

As chromium supplementation will often create a decreased need for insulin and other blood-glucose-lowering drugs used by type 1 and type 2 diabetics, it is recommended that individuals seeking to incorporate chromium into their treatment plan notify their doctor to prevent possible episodes of hypoglycemia.

Aloe Vera

Two preliminary trials found that aloe vera juice (containing 80 percent aloe gel) helps lower blood-sugar levels in people with type 2 diabetes. One trial found that one tablespoon (15 grams) twice daily reduced the amount of the blood-sugar-lowering drug glibenclamide. The other trial found that using the juice by itself was effective in lowering blood-sugar levels.

Essential Fatty Acids (EFAs)

Essential fatty acids also affect the ability of the body's cells to respond to insulin. In a 1993 study, Australian researchers learned that insulin resistance is related to the kinds of fatty acids that make up cell membranes. The more omega-3 and omega-6 fatty acids there are in the cell membranes of adult diabetics, the more easily their tissues respond to insulin.

Some diabetics seem to be blocked from converting short-chain omega-6 linoleic acid into the longer-chain acids needed for both cell membranes and prostaglandins. Noted researchers David Horrobin and Udo Erasmus are using supplements that contain omega-6 oil called gamma linolenic acid (GLA) to bypass the blocked processes. Damage to nerves, a big problem for many diabetics, has been halted or even reversed by GLA supplements.

Diabetics are not the only ones to receive benefits from essential fatty acid supplementation because deficiency creates symptoms in various and supposedly unconnected areas of the body.

EFA supplementation can benefit conditions such as premenstrual syndrome, scleroderma, eczema, and other skin conditions, with further investigation revealing that many individuals suffering from these and other conditions are not able to convert essential fatty acids into GLA. Consequently, evening primrose oil (EPO), which is naturally high in GLA, has helped in these conditions.

It has been theorized that a substantial portion of the population in the West is probably GLA deficient as a result of dietary deficiency, aging, high fat intake as well as glucose intolerance.

In most cases of long-term diabetes, a painful condition called diabetic neuropathy eventually occurs. A double-blind study reported dramatically improved nerve function and pain relief with the use of 4 grams of EPO per day for six months.

People with deficiencies would presumably benefit from supplemental GLA intake from EPO, black currant seed oil, or borage oil.

Gymnema Sylvestre

This indigenous Indian herb has been used in ayurvedic medicine for thousands of years. Gymnema leaves raise insulin levels, according to research in healthy volunteers. Based on animal studies, this may be due to regeneration of the cells in the pancreas that secrete insulin.

Gymnema works on several separate levels according to animal research; it improves the cells receptivity of glucose and at the same time stops the liver from producing and secreting glucose due to adrenaline stimulation, which then reduces overall blood-sugar levels.

Gymnemic acid is one possible constituent responsible for much of gymnema's activity. Gymnema also has been reported to lower cholesterol and triglyceride levels. Another curious characteristic is when Gymnema is taken orally, it blocks the taste of sweetness on the tongue, which may prove helpful to reduce cravings for sugars.

Banaba

Although this herb is a relative newcomer to natural medicine in the West, much research has been done on this particular plant and its ability to control blood sugar due to its primary insulin-like constituent, corosolic acid.

Most of the research into banaba has been done in Japan with many of these studies reporting astonishing properties associated with banaba.

The blood-sugar-regulating characteristics are effective even when the plant has been utilized once by another organism. An example of this would be a chicken experiment where chickens were fed banaba leaf powder and the egg yolks analyzed. The same egg yolks were then fed to diabetic mice with the end result of a normalization of blood sugar.

In another study, a mist containing extract of banaba was sprayed into the air where a diabetic patient lay sleeping. Trace amounts of corosolic acid was absorbed through the lungs, which then succeeded in regulating blood-sugar levels.

U.S. studies reported that corosolic acid lowers blood-sugar levels of all diabetic patients in a dose-dependent manner meaning the higher the dose, the lower the blood sugar.

However, more recent studies report that corosolic acid is probably not the only active ingredient in banaba leaves. A whole-leaf extract was studied in comparison to insulin activity and successfully treated diabetes and obesity.

Another recent study identified at least three other active components that improve glucose transport into cells, proving that corosolic acid was not the only active constituent found in banaba.

Fenugreek Seed

Fenugreek seeds are another example of an ayurvedic herb that has been used for thousands of years to treat diabetes. The seeds contain alkaloids and steroidal saponins as well as fiber, which collectively are thought to account for many of its medicinal properties and characteristics. The steroidal saponins are believed to inhibit cholesterol absorption and production while maintaining HDL cholesterol (the "good"cholesterol), while the fiber may help lower blood-sugar levels.

Several human studies have reported that fenugreek can assist in reducing cholesterol and triglycerides and help control blood-sugar levels in patients with atherosclerosis and type 2 diabetes and even help to a certain degree with insulin-dependent type 1 diabetes.

The dosage recommended by the German Commission E is 6 grams a day, however the dose needed to control diabetes or lower cholesterol is between 5 and 30 grams with each meal or 15 to 90 grams in a once-a-day dose taken with a meal. Fenugreek tincture is also effective at a dosage of 3 to 4 ml three times a day.

Glucomannan

Glucomannan is a fiber derived from the konjac root and has been traditionally used as a treatment for constipation. More recent research has revealed another side to this fiber. This slowing of the digestive process also increases the time it takes for sugars to enter the bloodstream, helping to control or slow the rise of blood-sugar levels.

This effect has been noted in studies where fiber was used in conjunction with a regular meal. Those utilizing this fiber exhibited lowered total blood-sugar levels in comparison to those who did not ingest glucomannan. It may also be helpful in cases of gestational diabetes as well as those with insulin resistance and metabolic syndrome.

Addition of relatively small amounts of glucomannan has prevented hypoglycemia in patients that have undergone stomach surgery, however studies in children had inconsistent results.

It has been theorized that glucomannan has the capability of reducing cholesterol and is thought to accomplish this by binding to bile acids and carrying them out of the body in bowel movements. This of course will force the body to change cholesterol into more bile acids to facilitate oil and fat digestion with the end result of cholesterol reduction.

This has been corroborated by several studies that reported significantly reduced cholesterol and triglyceride levels with the use of several grams per day of glucomannan even in patients with insulin-resistance syndrome.

Alpha Lipoic Acid

While alpha lipoic acid does little to help control blood-sugar levels, its powerful antioxidant properties have been used in Europe for decades to reduce the signs, symptoms, and pain of diabetic neuropathy. This painful condition is common in patients with long-standing diabetes and eventually leads to permanent nerve damage throughout the body.

Many studies have been done that prove that ALA will improve the sensitivity of insulin and slow the progression of kidney damage as well as reducing the signs of diabetic neuropathy in patients with either type 1 or type 2 diabetes. The average dose needed is 600 mg per day for eighteen months.

Magnesium

Human studies have indicated that insulin production in type 2 diabetic seniors is low, however supplementing with magnesium increases insulin production and secretion.

One double-blind study reported there was no beneficial effect with supplementation of 500 mg magnesium a day, but an increase of the magnesium dosage to 1,000 mg per day produced improvements.

Inconsistent results were reported from some double-blind studies that reported non-diabetic seniors can also produce more insulin with the use of magnesium supplements. According to other reports, the insulin dosage was reduced in type 1 senior diabetics with the use of magnesium, however a Dutch study reported there was no improvement in blood-sugar levels in people with type 2 diabetes. There seems to be a connection between magnesium deficiency and diabetic retinopathy.

Although there is normally a higher risk of spontaneous miscarriage and birth defects in diabetic pregnant women, pregnant women with magnesium deficiency have an even higher rate of spontaneous miscarriage and birth defects than pregnant women with sufficient magnesium levels and pregnant non-diabetic women; it has been theorized that magnesium supplementation may correct this situation.

Although the American Diabetes Association states that there are strong associations between insulin-resistant diabetes and magnesium deficiency, they will not definitively state that magnesium deficiency is a risk factor during pregnancy. Despite the ADA's reticence, many doctors suggest that pregnant women with diabetes with normal kidney function take 200 to 600 mg of magnesium per day to offset any possible deficiency.

Secondary Treatment Options

Cinnamon

Both herbs and spices appear to be beneficial in the treatment of diabetes. A study from the Tang-An Health Center in Beijing, China, examined the insulin-potentiating effects of cinnamon (*Cinnamonum mairei*), he shou wu (*Polygonum multiflorum*) and agaricus mushroom (*Agaricaceae*) in twenty-eight type 2 diabetics.

With the use of all three of these herbs, blood-glucose levels as well as total cholesterol during fasting were improved. Although cinnamon was not used alone, the positive results of this particular study were enough to initiate further investigations on cinnamon's potential effectiveness in treating diabetes.

One rat study done at Nagoya University in Japan reported that a cinnamon dose of 300 mg per kilo of body weight administered over three weeks increased insulin action on skeletal muscle and increased muscle absorption of blood sugar per minute by 17 percent.

In a human study in Pakistan, sixty people with type 2 diabetes were divided into six groups, receiving over forty days a placebo or 1 gram per day, 3 grams per day, or 6 grams per day of cinnamon. Cinnamon was found to reduce fasting serum glucose and cholesterol markers even in those participants that used only 1 gram of cinnamon per day. All three levels of cinnamon reduced blood-sugar levels by 18–29 percent, triglycerides 23–30 percent, LDL cholesterol 7–27 percent, and total cholesterol by 12–26 percent. This is an indication that cinnamon's effectiveness is dose dependent, meaning that the higher the dose the more effective it is, however even a low dosage such as 1 gram per day can be effective.

Studies initiated by the U.S. Department of Agriculture have attempted to identify the compound responsible in cinnamon for its blood-glucose modulating effect. The studies have been successful in identifying the compound as an A-type doubly linked procyanidin oligomer, which accounts for its strong antioxidant and glucose-controlling activity.

Vanadium

Studies involving vanadium in the form of vanadyl sulfate stated it may be effective in helping control blood glucose levels in type 2 diabetics; however type 1 diabetics did not respond nearly as well.

In a six-week double-blind human study, type 2 diabetics were given between 75 and 300 mg of vanadium in the form of vanadyl sulfate per day. The doses that were most effective in decreasing blood-sugar and sugar metabolism overall were in the 150 mg to 300 mg per day dosage, however improvements in insulin sensitivity were not noted.

At the 300 mg dosage level there was a decrease in cholesterol levels, which is beneficial; unfortunately HDL cholesterol (the "good" cholesterol) was also lowered.

One other side effect of vanadium supplementation was gastrointestinal upset, which was experienced by some of the participants using the 150 mg dose per day and by all of the participants using 300 mg per day. Due to this consequence, toxic reaction or side effects of long-term use of high-dose vanadium in doses exceeding 100 mg per day still need study as many physicians and researchers believe this dosage may be unsafe.

L- Carnitine

This conditionally essential amino acid is created by lysine and methionine in the body and is needed to transport fatty acids into cells for conversion into energy by the mitochondria. In situations of high energy expenditure such as pregnancy, athletic training and breastfeeding the need for L-carnitine can be lower than its production rate, creating a shortage.

Studies have reported that diabetics that were given L-carnitine at a dosage of 1 mg per kilo of body weight over ten days had as much as a 39 percent reduction in cholesterol and triglyceride levels. Injections of 1 gram per day of L-carnitine have reportedly reduced diabetic nerve pain and damage as well.

Diet and Prediabetes

We've all heard of the food pyramid that was initiated decades ago by the U.S. government. It may be that adherence to this outdated method of eating has partially contributed to the huge increase of diabetes in the West. In order to address this situation, the American Diabetes Association has created its own food pyramid. This new pyramid is substantially different from anything else, because whole grains, legumes, beans, and other high-fiber foods form the largest part or the base of the pyramid. By concentrating on high-fiber, low-glycemic-index, complex-carbohydrate foods such as oats and white beans, for example, while reducing or eliminating simple carbohydrates with high glycemic values, such a sugars and flours, it is hoped that a reduction in total blood glucose values will be realized by reducing insulin levels along with reduced blood cholesterol.

By decreasing or substituting meat with other foods such as brown rice or soy protein in recipes such as soups, stews, or casseroles, a reduction in saturated fats in the diet can be realized as well.

The smallest part of the pyramid at the top contains sweets, candies, desserts, alcohol, and fats or oils and should be eaten less often and in smaller servings.

Changes in margarine formulations and manufacturing have given us products that contain omega-3 fatty acids and plant sterols and are much more heart healthy when safely incorporated into a healthy diet. Not all fats and oils are unhealthy, but saturated and trans fats should be avoided at all costs. Substitute the unhealthy fats and oils with monounsaturated and polyunsaturated oils and oils that are generally high in omega-3 and omega-6 essential fatty acids such as olive oil.

Digestion

Digestion obviously plays a role in diabetes and food metabolism. The more efficient you are in breaking down, absorbing, and utilizing the nutrients in your diet, the less likely you are to have problems with deficiencies. Of course, this is assuming that you're eating the proper foods to begin with. In order to reduce stress and strain on the digestive organs, it is usually advised that:

· Four to six smaller meals are eaten per day rather than the more traditional three large meals
· Sufficient production of enzymes such as amylase helps to ensure efficient carbohydrate breakdown
· By ensuring that a regular supply of blood sugar is present and reducing blood-sugar spikes, you could reduce the incidence of carbohydrate cravings
· EFA consumption is crucial in maintaining the health

and viability of cell walls and in reducing the incidence
of insulin resistance or Syndrome X
· Significantly reduce or eliminate simple sugars in all
forms from your diet

The Importance of Fiber

A high-fiber diet has been shown to work better in controlling diabetes than the diet recommended by the ADA, and
may control blood-sugar levels as well as oral diabetes drugs.
In one study, the increase in dietary fiber was accomplished
exclusively through the consumption of foods naturally high in
fiber such as leafy green vegetables, granola, and fruit to a level
beyond that recommended by the ADA. No fiber supplements
were given. This six-week double-blind human study included
utilization of the ADA diet recommendations, which provided
24 grams of fiber per day along with an extra 50 grams of fiber
through the addition of other high-fiber foods. At the end of
the six-week test period the participants that ate only the ADA-
recommended diet had a blood-glucose level that was 10 percent higher than those participants who ate the ADA diet in
combination with the extra high-fiber foods. The high-fiber
participants also reported a 12 percent decrease in blood insulin levels as a result of increased insulin sensitivity. The high-
fiber participants also received the added benefit of significant
lowering of total cholesterol, triglycerides, and LDL, the "bad"
cholesterol.

Studies on specific fiber supplements derived from pectin,
guar gum, fenugreek seeds, and psyllium along with glucomannan have all improved blood glucose levels and for this reason
medical researchers and physicians all recommend a diet high
in fiber derived from fruits, whole grains, seeds, and oats, and
raw or steamed vegetables.

Protein and Carbohydrates

Many popular diets, such as the South Beach Diet, Sugar Busters, and the Atkins Diet, typically include high amounts of protein while restricting carbohydrates, especially refined sugars and flours. In some diets, there were unlimited calories and sometimes unlimited fat, and many books were written to guide new acolytes to the ultimate weight-loss secret.

We all know that carbohydrates affect blood-sugar and insulin levels and for this reason advocates of the high-protein diet believe that carbohydrates should be avoided or dramatically reduced to decrease insulin release, which can cause insulin to store extra fats. They believe that high protein and fat consumption does not contribute to weight gain as they do not increase blood-sugar or insulin secretion. Recommended carbohydrates that are included in high-protein diets include fruits, fiber-containing grains, and vegetables.

Although high-protein diets have come under scrutiny in the past years, recent studies have reported positive results or at least a lack of negative consequences from adherence to high-protein, low carbohydrate diets.

In spite of this, the United States Department of Agriculture's revised Food Guide Pyramid still calls for six to eleven servings of carbohydrate foods such as flours, bread, cereal, rice, and pasta each day. It is no wonder that obesity is in the top three medical issues facing North Americans today.

As long as we insist on taking in more calories than we expend every day through exercise and metabolism, we cannot help but set off a cascade of unhealthy physiological events that will result in weight gain, high blood pressure, and elevated cholesterol, along with a dramatically increased risk of metabolic syndrome and type 2 diabetes.

Glycemic Index

The glycemic index ranks carbohydrates based on their immediate effect on blood-sugar levels. The faster a food increases blood-sugar levels, the higher the glycemic index. An example of a high-glycemic food would be sugar and low-glycemic foods would be celery and oats because these foods digest slowly, consequently releasing their sugars more gradually into the bloodstream.

How quickly carbohydrates are converted into sugars is determined by other foods that are eaten along with the carbohydrate, the amount of fiber in the carbohydrate, and how well your digestive system works. As we age, the digestive system reduces activity, which increases the length of time it takes for digestion to occur. It is safe to say that in general, high-fiber foods have a reduced effect on blood sugars and therefore can be considered to be low glycemic in nature.

The glycemic index runs from 0 to 100 in accordance to how quickly and how high the food increases blood-sugar levels. You may be shocked to realize what foods are included in the high-glycemic list. This list contains most breakfast cereals, breads, and, surprisingly, baked potatoes, which have a glycemic index much greater than sugar. Considering that potatoes are the most frequently eaten vegetable in the Western world, this should be of great concern.

High Glycemic Value foods include:
- Baked potatoes
- Corn flakes
- Ice cream
- Instant oatmeal
- Mashed potatoes
- French fries
- Couscous

Low glycemic foods include:
- Beans
- Barley
- Pasta
- Oats
- Some types of rice
- Acidic fruits
- Vinegar and lemon juice

What is glycemic load?

This is a recently developed method that incorporates not only the glycemic index of the food but also how much carbohydrate is contained in a typical serving size. This method gives a fuller and more accurate view of the impact particular foods have on blood sugar.

The carbohydrate in watermelon, for example, has a high GI, meaning that it has a strong effect on blood sugar, however there isn't a lot of carbohydrate found in watermelon for each serving. Consequently watermelon's glycemic load is not particularly high.

Conclusion

You can do more than you ever imagined to treat your diabetes and prediabetes. Even if there is a genetic predisposition, it does not mean that you are doomed to develop full-blown diabetes; however you must take full responsibility, educate yourself, and exercise discipline. If you use even half of the information in this book, you will not only dramatically reduce your chances of developing a blood-sugar condition, you can successfully treat it yourself using natural, safe, and effective methods. Reading this book and being willing to change is 50 percent of your journey and future success.

In order to gain the best benefit from this information, it is not enough to simply take these or other supplements in an attempt to control your blood sugar. Dietary choices are a primary driving force behind diabetes, so you must be willing to make lifestyle and dietary changes in order to gain the most from your effort to control your prediabetic condition. These strategies work, but you'll only get the results you want with discipline and consistent work.

References

Abraira C, Derler J. Large variations of sucrose in constant carbohydrate diets in type 2 diabetes. *Am J Med* 1988;84:193–200.

American Diabetes Association. Magnesium supplementation in the treatment of diabetes. *Diabetes Care* 1992;15:1065–7.

American Diabetes Association. Position Statement: nutrition recommendations and principles for people with diabetes mellitus. *Diabetes Care* 1999;22:S42–5 [review].

Anderson RA, Cheng N, Bryden NA, et al. Elevated intakes of supplemental chromium improve glucose and insulin variables in individuals with type 2 diabetes. *Diabetes* 1997;46:1786–91.

Anderson RA, Polansky MM, Bryden NA, Canary JJ. Supplemental-chromium effects on glucose, insulin, glucagon, and urinary chromium losses in subjects consuming controlled low-chromium diets. *Am J Clin Nutr* 1991;54:909–16.

Anderson RA, Polansky MM, Bryden NA, et al. Chromium supplementation of human subjects: effects on glucose, insulin, and lipid variables. *Metabolism* 1983;32:894–9.

Anderson RA. Chromium in the prevention and control of diabetes. *Diabetes Metab* 2000;26:22–7 [review].

Anderson RA. Chromium, glucose intolerance and diabetes. *J Am Coll Nutr* 1998;17:548–55 [review].

Arvill A, Bodin L. Effect of short-term ingestion of konjac glucomannan on serum cholesterol in healthy men. *Am J Clin Nutr* 1995;61:585–9.

Baba NH, Sawaya S, Torbay N, et al. High protein vs high carbohydrate hypoenergetic diet for the treatment of obese hyperinsulinemic subjects. *Int J Obes Relat Metab Disord* 1999;23:1202–6.

Bishayee A, Chatterjee M. Hypolipidemic and antiatherosclerotic effects of oral Gymnema sylvestre R.Br. leaf extract in albino rats fed on a high fat diet. *Phytother Res* 1994;8:118–20.

Blumenthal M, Busse WR, Goldberg A, et al. (eds). The Complete Commission E Monographs: Therapeutic Guide to Herbal Medicines. Boston: Integrative Medicine Communications, 1998, 130.

Bordia A, Verma SK, Srivastava KC. Effect of ginger (Zingiber officinale Rosc) and fenugreek (Trigonella foenumgraecum L) on blood lipids, blood sugar, and platelet aggregation in patients with coronary artery disease. *Prostagland Leukotrienes Essential Fatty Acids* 1997;56:379–84.

Brand-Miller J, Foster-Powell K. Diets with a low glycemic index: from theory to practice. *Nutr Today* 1999;34:64–72 [review].

Bunyapraphatsara N, Yongchaiyudha S, Rungpitarangsi V, Chokechaijaroenporn O. Antidiabetic activity of *Aloe vera* L juice II. Clinical trial in diabetes mellitus patients in combination with glibenclamide. *Phytomedicine* 1996;3:245–8.

Carper, Jean. *Stop Aging Now!* (New York: 1995, Harper Perennial, a division of Harper Collin Publishers), pages 81 and 307. ISBN 0-06-018355-1

Cesa F, Mariani S, Fava A, et al. The use of vegetable fibers in the treatment of pregnancy diabetes and/or excessive weight gain during pregnancy. *Minerva Ginecol* 1990;42:271–4 [in Italian].

Chandalia M, Garg A, Lutjohann D, et al. Beneficial effects of high dietary fiber intake in patients with type 2 diabetes mellitus. *New Engl J Med* 2000;342:1392–8.

Cohen AM, Bavly S, Poznanski R. Change of diet of Yemenite Jews in relation to diabetes and ischaemic heart-disease. *Lancet* 1961;2:1399–401.

Cohen AM, Fidel J, Cohen B, et al. Diabetes, blood lipids, lipoproteins, and change of environment: restudy of the "new immigrant Yemenites" in Israel. *Metabolism* 1979;28:716–28.

Cohen D, Dodds R, Viberti G. Effect of protein restriction in insulin dependent diabetics at risk of nephropathy. *BMJ* 1987;294:795–8.

Colagiuri S, Miller JJ, Edwards RA. Metabolic effects of adding sucrose and aspartame to the diet of subjects with noninsulin-dependent diabetes mellitus. *Am J Clin Nutr* 1989;50:474–8.

Colditz GA, Manson JE, Stampfer MJ, et al. Diet and risk of clinical diabetes in women. *Am J Clin Nutr* 1992;55:1018–23.

Colgan, Ph.D., Michael, *The New Nutrition: Medicine for the New Millennium* (Vancouver: 1995, Apple Publishing), pages 10-11. ISBN 0-9695272-4-1

Cooper, M.D., M.P.H., Kenneth H. *Advanced Nutritional Therapies* (Nashville: 1996, Thomas Nelson, Inc. Publishers), pages 165-166.

Crane MG, Sample C. Regression of diabetic neuropathy with total vegetarian (vegan) diet. *J Nutr Med* 1994;4:431–9.

Crane MG, Sample CJ. Regression of diabetic neuropathy with vegan diet. *Am J Clin Nutr* 1988;48:926 [abstract #P28].

de Valk HW, Verkaaik R, van Rijn HJM, et al. Oral magnesium supplementation in insulin-requiring type 2 diabetic patients. *Diabet Med* 1998;15:503–7.

Diabetes Atlas, Second Edition, International Diabetes Federation, 2003.

Doi K, Matsuura M, Kawara A, Baba S. Treatment of diabetes with glucomannan (konjac mannan). *Lancet* 1979;1:987–8 [letter].

Doi K. Effect of konjac fibre (glucomannan) on glucose and lipids. *Eur J Clin Nutr* 1995;49(Suppl. 3):S190–7 [review].

Donaghue KC, Pena MM, Chan AK, et al. Beneficial effects of increasing monounsaturated fat intake in adolescents with type 1 diabetes. *Diabetes Res Clin Pract* 2000;48:193–9.

Eibl NL, Schnack CJ, Kopp H-P, et al. Hypomagnesemia in type 2 diabetes: effect of a 3-month replacement therapy. *Diabetes Care* 1995;18:188.

Evanoff G, Thompson C, Bretown J, Weinman E. Prolonged dietary protein restriction in diabetic nephropathy. *Arch Intern Med* 1989;149:1129–33.

Evans GW. The effect of chromium picolinate on insulin controlled parameters in humans. *Int J Biosocial Med Res* 1989;11:163–80.

Feskens EJ, Bowles CH, Kromhout D. Carbohydrate intake and body mass index in relation to the risk of glucose intolerance in an elderly population. *Am J Clin Nutr* 1991;54:136–40.

Feskens EJ, Bowles CH, Kromhout D. Carbohydrate intake and body mass index in relation to the risk of glucose intolerance in an elderly population. *Am J Clin Nutr* 1991;54:136–40.

Feskens EJ, Kromhout D. Habitual dietary intake and glucose tolerance in euglycaemic men: the Zutphen Study. *Int J Epidemiol* 1990;19:953–9.

Feskens EJ, Virtanen SM, Rasanen L, et al. Dietary factors determining diabetes and impaired glucose tolerance. A 20-year follow-up of the Finnish and Dutch cohorts of the Seven Countries Study. *Diabetes Care* 1995;18:1104–12.

Feskens EJM, Bowles CH, Kromhout D. Inverse association between fish intake and risk of glucose intolerance in normoglycemic elderly men and women. *Diabetes Care* 1991;14:935–41.

Florholmen J, Arvidsson-Lenner R, Jorde R, Burhol PG. The effect of Metamucil on postprandial blood glucose and plasma gastric inhibitory peptide in insulin-dependent diabetics. *Acta Med Scand* 1982;212:237–9.

Forbes S, Bui S, Robinson BR, Hochgeschwender U, Brennan MB. Integrated control of appetite and fat metabolism by the leptin-proopiomelanocortin pathway. *Proc Natl Acad Sci U S A.* 2001 Mar 27;98(7):4233-7.

Fushiki T, Kojima A, Imoto T, et al. An extract of Gymnema sylvestre leaves and purified gymnemic acid inhibits glucose-stimulated gastric inhibitory peptide secretion in rats. *J Nutr* 1992;122: 2367–73.

Gaby AR, Wright JV. Diabetes. In *Nutritional Therapy in Medical Practice: Reference Manual and Study Guide.* Kent, WA: 1996, 54–64 [review].

Gaby AR, Wright JV. Nutritional protocols: diabetes mellitus. In *Nutritional Therapy in Medical Practice: Protocols and Supporting Information.* Kent, WA: 1996, 10.

Garg A, Bananome A, Grundy SM, et al. Comparison of a high-carbohydrate diet with a high-monounsaturated-fat diet in patients with non-insulin dependent diabetes mellitus. *N Engl J Med* 1988;319:829–34.

Gin H, Aparicio M, Potauz L, et al. Low-protein, low-phosphorus diet and tissue insulin sensitivity in insulin-dependent diabetic patients with chronic renal failure. *Nephron* 1991;57:411–5.

Glen AIM, Glen EMT, MacDonnell LEF, et al. Essential fatty acids in the management of withdrawal symptoms and tissue damage in alcoholics, presented at the 2nd International Congress on Essential Fatty Acids, Prostaglandins and Leukotrienes, London, Zoological Society. March 24–7, 1985,

Gymnema monograph. *Lawrence Review of Natural Products.* Aug 1993.

Hattori K et al. "Activation of insulin receptors by lagerstroemin." *J Pharmacol Sci.* 93, 1:69-73, 2003.

Herepath WB. *Journal Provincial Med Surg Soc* 1854:374.

Hermann J, Chung H, Arquitt A, et al. Effects of chromium or copper supplementation on plasma lipids, plasma glucose and serum insulin in adults over age fifty. *J Nutr Elderly* 1998;18:27–45.

Hopman WP, Houben PG, Speth PA, Lamers CB. Glucomannan prevents postprandial hypoglycaemia in patients with previous gastric surgery. *Gut* 1988;29:930–4.

Horrobin DF, Campbell A. Sjogren's syndrome and the sicca syndrome: the role of prostaglandin E1 deficiency. Treatment with essential fatty acids and vitamin C. *Med Hypotheses* 1980;6:225–32.

Horrobin DF, Manku M, Brush M, et al. Abnormalities in plasma essential fatty acid levels in women with pre-menstrual syndrome and with non-malignant breast disease. *J Nutr Med* 1991;2:259–64.

Horrobin DF. Essential fatty acid metabolism in diseases of connective tissue with special reference to scleroderma and to Sjogren's syndrome. *Med Hypotheses* 1984;14:233–47.

Horrobin DF. Essential fatty acids in clinical dermatology. *J Am Acad Dermatol* 1989;20:1045–53.

Huang CY, Zhang MY, Peng SS, et al. Effect of Konjac food on blood glucose level in patients with diabetes. *Biomed Environ Sci* 1990;3:123–31.

Jamal GA, Carmichael H. The effect of gamma-linolenic acid on human diabetic peripheral neuropathy: a double-blind placebo-controlled trial.*Diabet Med* 1990;7:319-23

Jovanovic L, Gutierrez M, Peterson CM. Chromium supplementation for women with gestational diabetes. *J Trace Elem Exptl Med* 1999; 12:91–8.

Kakuda T, Sakane I, Takihara T, Ozaki Y, Takeuchi H, Kuroyanagi M. Hypoglycemic effect of extracts from Lagerstroemia speciosa L. leaves in genetically diabetic KK-AY mice. *Biosci Biotechnol Biochem.* 1996 Feb;60(2):204-8.

Keen H, Payan J, Allawi J, et al. Treatment of diabetic neuropathy with gamma-linolenic acid. *Diabetes Care* 1993;16:8–15.

Klatz, D.O., Ronald and Goldman, D.O., Robert. *Stopping the Clock* (New Canaan, Connecticut: Keats Publishing, Inc., 1996), pages 112 and 115. ISBN: 0-87983-717-9

Kneepkens CM, Fernandes J, Vonk RJ. Dumping syndrome in children. Diagnosis and effect of glucomannan on glucose tolerance and absorption. *Acta Paediatr Scand* 1988;77:279–86.

Konrad T, Vicini P, Kusterer K, et al. Apha lipoic acid treatment decreases serum lactate and pyruvate concentrations and improves glucose effectiveness in lean and obese patients with type 2 diabetes. *Diabetes Care* 1999; 22:280–7.

Landin K, Holm G, Tengborn L, Smith U. Guar gum improves insulin sensitivity, blood lipids, blood pressure, and fibrinolysis in healthy men. *Am J Clin Nutr* 1992;56:1061–5.

Lee NA, Reasner CA. Beneficial effect of chromium supplementation on serum triglyceride levels in NIDDM. *Diabetes Care* 1994;17:1449–52.

Lempiainen P, Mykkanen L, Pyorala K, et al. Insulin resistance syndrome predicts coronary heart disease events in elderly nondiabetic men. *Circulation* 1999;100:123–8.

Liese AD, Mayer-Davis EJ, Haffner SM. Development of the insulin resistance syndrome: an epidemiologic perspective. *Epidemiol Rev* 1998;20:157–72.

Lima M, Cruz T, Carreiro Pousada J, et al: The effect of magnesium supplementation in increasing doses on the control of type 2 diabetes. *Diabetes Care* 1998;21:682–6.

Liu F et al. "An extract of Lagerstroemia speciosa L. has insulin-like glucose uptake-stimulatory and adipocyte differentiation-inhibitory activities in 3T3-L1 cells." *J Nutr*. 131, 9:2242-7, 2001

Loghmani E, Rickard K, Washburne L, et al. Glycemic response to sucrose-containing mixed meals in diets of children with insulin-dependent diabetes mellitus. *J Pediatr* 1991;119:531–7.

Madar Z, Abel R, Samish S, Arad J. Glucose-lowering effect of fenugreek in non-insulin dependent diabetics. *Eur J Clin Nutr* 1988;42:51–4.

Manku MS, Horrobin, DF, Morse NL, et al. Essential fatty acids in the plasma phospholipids of patients with atopic eczema. *Br J Derm* 1984;110:643.

Mansel RE, Pye JK, Hughes LE. Effects of essential fatty acids on cyclical mastalgia and noncyclical breast disorders. In Omega-6 Essential Fatty Acids: Pathophysiology and Roles in Clinical Medicine, ed. DF Horrobin. New York: Alan R Liss, 1990, 557–66.

Marshall JA, Hamman RF, Baxter J. High-fat, low-carbohydrate diet and the etiology of non-insulin-dependent diabetes mellitus: the San Luis Valley Diabetes Study. *Am J Epidemiol* 1991;134:590–603.

Marshall JA, Hoag S, Shetterly S, et al. Dietary fat predicts conversion from impaired glucose tolerance to NIDDM. The San Luis Valley Diabetes Study. *Diabetes Care* 1994;17:50–6.

McNair P, Christiansen C, Madsbad S, et al. Hypomagnesemia, a risk factor in diabetic retinopathy. *Diabetes* 1978;27:1075–7.

Melga P, Giusto M, Ciuchi E, et al. Dietary fiber in the dietetic therapy of diabetes mellitus. Experimental data with purified glucomannans. *Riv Eur Sci Med Farmacol* 1992;14:367–73 [in Italian].

Mhasker KS, Caius JF. A study of Indian medicinal plants. II. Gymnema sylvestre R.Br. *Indian J Med Res Memoirs* 1930;16:2–75.

Mimouni F, Miodovnik M, Tsang RC, et al. Decreased maternal serum magnesium concentration and adverse fetal outcome in insulin-dependent diabetic women. *Obstet Gynecol* 1987;70:85–9.

Moore MA, Park CB, Tsuda H. Implications of the hyperinsulinaemia-diabetes-cancer link for preventive efforts. *Eur J Cancer Prev* 1998;7:89–107 [review].

Morcos M, Borcea V, Isermann B, et al. Effect of alpha-lipoic acid on the progression of endothelial cell damage and albuminuria in patients with diabetes mellitus: an exploratory study. *Diabetes Res Clin Pract* 2001;52:175–83.

Mori TA, Bao DQ, Burke V, et al. Dietary fish as a major component of a weight-loss diet: effect on serum lipids, glucose, and insulin metabolism in overweight hypertensive subjects. *Am J Clin Nutr* 1999;70:817–25.

Nuttall FW. Dietary fiber in the management of diabetes. *Diabetes* 1993;42:503–8.

Offenbacher EG, Pi-Sunyer FX. Beneficial effect of chromium-rich yeast on glucose tolerance and blood lipids in elderly subjects. *Diabetes* 1980;29:919–25.

Paolisso G, Scheen A, D'Onofrio FD, Lefebvre P. Magnesium and glucose homeostasis. *Diabetologia* 1990;33:511–4 [review].

Paolisso G, Sgambato S, Gambardella A, et al. Daily magnesium supplements improve glucose handling in elderly subjects. *Am J Clin Nutr* 1992;55:1161–7.

Paolisso G, Sgambato S, Pizza G, et al. Improved insulin response and action by chronic magnesium administration in aged NIDDM subjects. *Diabetes Care* 1989;12:265–9.

Popkin B, S Nelson. The sweetening of the world's diet. Obesity Research; 11: pp 1325-1332 November 2003.

Prasanna M. Hypolipidemic effect of fenugreek: A clinical study. *Indian J Phramcol* 2000;32:34–6.

Pyorala M, Miettinen H, Halonen P, et al. Insulin resistance syndrome predicts the risk of coronary heart disease and stroke in healthy middle-aged men: the 22-year follow-up results of the Helsinki Policemen Study. *Arterioscler Thromb Vasc Biol* 2000;20:538–44.

Rabinowitz MB, Gonick HC, Levin SR, Davidson MB. Effects of chromium and yeast supplements on carbohydrate and lipid metabolism in diabetic men. *Diabetes Care* 1983;6:319–27.

Raghuram TC, Sharma RD, Sivakumar B, Sahay BK. Effect of fenugreek seeds on intravenous glucose disposition in non-insulin dependent diabetic patients. *Phytother Res* 1994;8:83–6.

Reiser S, Hallfrisch J, Fields M, et al. Effects of sugars on indices of glucose tolerance in humans. *Am J Clin Nutr* 1986;43:151–9.

Reljanovic M, Reichel G, Rett K, et al. Treatment of diabetic polyneuropathy with the antioxidant thioctic acid (alpha-lipoic acid): a two year multicenter randomized double-blind placebo-controlled trial (ALADIN II). Alpha Lipoic Acid in Diabetic Neuropathy. *Free Radic Res* 1999;31:171–9.

Ribes G, Sauvaire Y, Da Costa C, et al. Antidiabetic effects of subfractions from fenugreek seeds in diabetic dogs. *Proc Soc Exp Biol Med* 1986;182:159–66.

Rodríguez-Morán M, Guerrero-Romero F, Lazcano-Burciaga G. Lipid- and glucose-lowering efficacy of plantago psyllium in type 2 diabetes. *Diabetes Its Complications* 1998;12:273–8.

Ruhnau KJ, Meissner HP, Finn JR, et al. Effects of 3-week oral treatment with the antioxidant thioctic acid (alpha-lipoic acid) in symptomatic diabetic polyneuropathy. *Diabet Med* 1999;16:1040–3.

Ruhnau KJ, Meissner HP, Finn JR, et al. Effects of 3-week oral treatment with the antioxidant thioctic acid (alpha-lipoic acid) in symptomatic diabetic polyneuropathy. *Diabet Med* 1999;16:1040–3.

Salmeron J, Manson JE, Stampfer MJ, et al. Dietary fiber, glycemic load, and risk of non-insulin-dependent diabetes mellitus in women. *JAMA* 1997;277:472–7.

Sarkkinen E, Schwab U, Niskanen L, et al. The effects of monounsaturated-fat enriched diet and polyunsaturated-fat enriched diet on lipid and glucose metabolism in subjects with impaired glucose tolerance. *Eur J Clin Nutr* 1996;50:592–8.

Sauvaire Y, Ribes G, Baccou JC, Loubatieres-Mariani MM. Implication of steroid saponins and sapogenins in the hypocholesterolemic effect of fenugreek. *Lipids* 1991;26:191–7.

Schalin-Karrila M, Mattila L, Jansen CT, et al. Evening primrose oil in the treatment of atopic eczema: effect on clinical status, plasma phospholipid fatty acids and circulating blood prostaglandins. *Br J Dermatol* 1987;117:11–9.

Schwartz SE, Levine RA, Weinstock RS, et al. Sustained pectin ingestion: effect on gastric emptying and glucose tolerance in non-insulin-dependent diabetic patients. *Am J Clin Nutr* 1988;48:1413–7.

Shanmugasundaram ER, Gopinath KL, Radha Shanmugasundaram K, Rajendran VM. Possible regeneration of the islets of Langerhans in streptozotocin diabetic rats given Gymnema sylvestre leaf extracts. *J Ethnopharmacol* 1990;30:265–79.

Shanmugasundaram KR, Panneerselvam C, Sumudram P, Shanmugasundaram ERB. Insulinotropic activity of G. sylvestre, R.Br. and Indian medicinal herb used in controlling diabetes mellitus. *Pharmacol Res Commun* 1981;13:475–86.

Sharma RD, Raghuram TC, Rao NS. Effect of fenugreek seeds on blood glucose and serum lipids in type 1 diabetes. *Eur J Clin Nutr* 1990;44:301–6.

Sharma RD, Raghuram TC. Hypoglycaemic effect of fenugreek seeds in non-insulin dependent diabetic subjects. *Nutr Res* 1990; 10: 731–9.

Sharma RD, Sarkar DK, Hazra B, et al. Hypolipidaemic effect of fenugreek seeds: A chronic study in non-insulin dependent diabetic patients. *Phytother Res* 1996;10:332–4.

Sherman L, Glennon JA, Brech WJ, et al. Failure of trivalent chromium to improve hyperglycemia in diabetes mellitus. *Metabolism* 1968;17:439–42.

Sjorgren A, Floren CH, Nilsson A. Oral administration of magnesium hydroxide to subjects with insulin dependent diabetes mellitus. *Magnesium* 1988;121:16–20.

Snowdon DA, Phillips RL. Does a vegetarian diet reduce the occurrence of diabetes? *Am J Publ Health* 1985;75:507–12.

Stoll BA. Western nutrition and the insulin resistance syndrome: a link to breast cancer. *Eur J Clin Nutr* 1999;53:83–7 [review].

Trevisan M, Liu J, Bahsas FB, Menotti A. Syndrome X and mortality: a population-based study. *Am J Epidemiol* 1998;148:958–66.

Tuomilehto Jaakko, M.D., Ph.D., Jaana Lindstrom, M.S., Johan G. Eriksson, M.D., Ph.D., Timo T. Valle, M.D. et. al. Prevention of type 2 Diabetes Mellitus by Changes in Lifestyle among Subjects with Impaired Glucose Tolerance. New Engl J Med May 3 2001 Volume 344:1343-1350

Urberg M, Zemel MB. Evidence for synergism between chromium and nicotinic acid in the control of glucose tolerance in elderly humans. *Metabolism* 1987;36:896–9.

Uusitupa M, Schwab U, Makimattila S, et al. Effects of two high-fat diets with different fatty acid compositions on glucose and lipid metabolism in healthy young women. *Am J Clin Nutr* 1994;59:1310–6.

Uusitupa MI, Kumpulainen JT, Voutilainen E, et al. Effect of inorganic chromium supplementation on glucose tolerance, insulin response, and serum lipids in noninsulin-dependent diabetics. *Am J Clin Nutr* 1983;38:404–10.

Vaddadi KS, Gilleard CJ. Essential fatty acids, tardive dyskinesia, and schizophrenia. In *Omega-6 Essential Fatty Acids: Pathophysiology and Roles in Clinical Medicine*, ed. DF Horrobin. New York: Alan R Liss, 1990, 333–43.

Vaddadi KS, Gilleard CJ. Essential fatty acids, tardive dyskinesia, and schizophrenia. In Omega-6 Essential Fatty Acids: Pathophysiology and Roles in Clinical Medicine. Horrobin DF (ed). New York: Alan R Liss, 1990, 333–43.

Valdez R. Epidemiology. *Nutr Rev* 2000;58:S4–S6 [review].

Vanhala MJ, Pitkajarvi TK, Kumpusalo EA, Takala JK. Obesity type and clustering of insulin resistance-associated cardiovascular risk factors in middle-aged men and women. *Int J Obes Relat Metab Disord* 1998;22:369–74.

Vorster HH, Lotter AP, Odendaal I, et al. Benefits from supplementation of the current recommended diabetic diet with gel fibre. *Int Clin Nutr Rev* 1988;8:140–6.

Vuksan V, Jenkins DJ, Spadafora P, et al. Konjac-mannan (glucomannan) improves glycemia and other associated risk factors for coronary heart disease in type 2 diabetes. A randomized controlled metabolic trial. *Diabetes Care* 1999;22:913–9.

Vuksan V, Jenkins DJ, Spadafora P, et al. Konjac-mannan (glucomannan) improves glycemia and other associated risk factors for coronary heart disease in type 2 diabetes. A randomized controlled metabolic trial. *Diabetes Care* 1999;22:913–9.

Vuksan V, Sievenpiper JL, Owen R, et al. Beneficial effects of viscous dietary fiber from Konjac-mannan in subjects with the insulin resistance syndrome: results of a controlled metabolic trial. *Diabetes Care* 2000;23:9–14.

Walsh DE, Yaghoubian V, Behforooz A. Effect of glucomannan on obese patients: a clinical study. *Int J Obes* 1984;8:289–93.

Wright DW, Hansen RI, Mondon CE, Reaven GM. Sucrose-induced insulin resistance in the rat: modulation by exercise and diet. *Am J Clin Nutr* 1983;38:879–83.

Wu J, Peng SS. Comparison of hypolipidemic effect of refined konjac meal with several common dietary fibers and their mechanisms of action. *Biomed Environ Sci* 1997;10:27–37.

www.cdc.gov/nchs/data/series/sr_10/sr10_222.pdf

www.healthpolitics.com/media/diabetes/slides

Yip J, Facchini FS, Reaven GM. Resistance to insulin-mediated glucose disposal as a predictor of cardiovascular disease. *J Clin Endocrinol Metab* 1998;83:2773–6.

Yongchaiyudha S, Rungpitarangsi V, Bunyapraphatsara N, Chokeshaijaroenporn O. Antidiabetic activity of *Aloe vera* L juice I. Clinical trial in new cases of diabetes mellitus. *Phytomedicine* 1996;3:241–3.

Zhang MY, Huang CY, Wang X, et al. The effect of foods containing refined Konjac meal on human lipid metabolism. *Biomed Environ Sci* 1990;3:99–105.

Ziegler D, Hanefeld M, Ruhnau KJ, et al. Treatment of symptomatic diabetic polyneuropathy with the antioxidant alpha-lipoic acid: a 7-month multicenter randomized controlled trial (ALADIN III Study). ALADIN III Study Group. Alpha-Lipoic Acid in Diabetic Neuropathy. *Diabetes Care* 1999;22:1296–301.

Ziegler D, Schatz H, Conrad F, et al. Effects of treatment with the antioxidant alpha-lipoic acid on cardiac autonomic neuropathy in NIDDM patients. A 4-month randomized controlled multicenter trial (DEKAN Study). *Diabetes Care* 1997;20:369–73.